Get Rid of the Blues

Everything You Always Wanted to Know
About Varicose and "Spider" Veins
But Didn't Know Who to Ask

Mary T. Johnson, RN

toExcel
San Jose New York Lincoln Shanghai

Get Rid of the Blues
Everything You Always Wanted to Know About Varicose and "Spider"
Veins But Didn't Know Who to Ask

Published by toExcel
an imprint of iUniverse.com, Inc.

For information address:
iUniverse.com, Inc.
620 North 48th Street
Suite 201
Lincoln, NE 68504-3467
www.iuniverse.com

The author gratefully acknowledges the support of Beiersdorf-Jobst, Inc.
(Manufacturers of JOBST® brand gradient support hosiery and socks) for
providing illustrations which appear within this book.

ISBN: 0-595-01074-1

Printed in the United States of America

Table of Contents

Acknowledgments

I'm very grateful to several people for sharing their time and expertise. I'd like to express special gratitude to Alan H. Kanter, MD for generously agreeing to be my medical editor and patient teacher, and for the countless hours he spent making sure I got it right. Many people will benefit because of his willingness to share the same level of commitment and ethics to this project that he brings to his practice and his research.

Mitchel P. Goldman, MD, Assistant Clinical Professor of Dermatology at the University of California, San Diego, has written extensively about venous disease and I appreciate his gracious efforts to clear up my questions on venous ulcers.

Thanks to Wayne M. Marley, MD, past president of the North American Society of Phlebology for his insights on vein disease in men.

I also wish to acknowlege Jorge Nieri, Senior Product Manager for Beiersdorf-Jobst, Inc. and D. Bruce Guynn, General Manager of Medi USA for helping me understand the manufacturing process for graduated compression. In addition, I am indebted to Mr. Nieri and Susan J. Sigman for their generous efforts to help me obtain illustrations for this book.

Additionally, I'd like to thank Gary Begley, President of National Laser Laboratories, Inc., for the technical information he provided on laser.

I am very grateful to Ruth Ann Wolfhope for generously agreeing to share the dramatic before and after photos of her legs.

And to Joe Baker, former Business Editor of the San Bernardino County Sun, thank you for putting on your editor's cap once again.

Book design and typography Cutter's Way Graphics.

About the Author

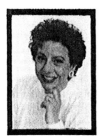 Mary T. Johnson, a registered nurse since 1982, began specializing in small vein disease in 1991. She was one of the first RNs in California to contract with physicians to offer sclerotherapy treatments (tiny injections into diseased veins) to their patients. Since then, she has served as a consultant and trains registered nurses to do sclerotherapy utilizing a training program she developed which has been approved for continuing education credit by the California State Board of Registered Nursing, and by the California Department of Rehabilitation for RN retraining. In 1993 she founded the National Association of Nurse Sclerotherapists and serves as the organization's executive director. She is also a member of the Society for Vascular Nursing and the American Medical Writers Association.

The author has written about varicose vein disease for the *Journal of Vascular Nursing* and has served as a contributing editor for *Your Family's Health Magazine*.

The author welcomes the opportunity to work with businesses, associations, and nonprofit organizations. Requests for availability for speeches and seminars, book signings, and participation in fund raisers should be directed to her at the address below. Readers of this book are also encouraged to contact the author at the address below with comments and ideas for future editions.

Mary T. Johnson
13537 Mesa Verde Dr.
Yucaipa CA 92399
E-Mail: scribe123@email.msn.com

Foreword

Varicose and spider veins affect the majority of people over the age of 50 worldwide, and many younger. Besides cosmetic embarrassment, they can cause uncomfortable symptoms, as well as potentially serious complications. It is therefore surprising that medical school curricula do not educate physicians on this all-too-common malady. By the time patients present with complications such as blood clots or leg ulcers, they are likely to have suffered years of needless discomfort, inconvenience, and probably misdirected neglect from those ignorant in its diagnosis and treatment. Fortunately, this sad situation is slowly changing.

Quantum leaps forward have occurred in the field of "phlebology" (venous disorders) during the last decade. Risk-free, out-patient duplex ultrasound has replaced in-patient x-ray procedures for diagnosis. Refinements have been made to both traditional methods of vein treatment (surgery and sclerotherapy) that render them safer, less expensive, more convenient, and more effective. In addition, light sources including lasers are just now emerging as a third treatment option for some vein conditions. And yet, where can the average person look for an objective, up-to-date discussion of these trends?

Many primary care physicians are reluctant to refer their patients for consultation for vein disease due to either managed-care financial constraints, simple ignorance of the problem, or perhaps the lack of a local source of reliable information. One finds that myths, anecdotes, and undocumented dogma abound surrounding vein disease. Except for small brochures from some professional specialty societies that briefly review the basics, notwithstanding the perennial onslaught of media hype, there is no unbiased source of information readily available to the public regarding vein disease.

Ms. Johnson has performed a long-overdue service in undertaking the writing of this book. After years of experience with physicians specializing in phlebology, she developed and implemented the first continuing education course in vein disease approved by the California State Board of Registered Nurses. After so educating her peers, she perceived the need for a more detailed reference to enable laypersons to make informed choices regarding the fate of their vein disease: preventative measures, whether and when to consider treatment, where to go for competent evaluation, and what to expect before, during, and after treatment.

As a practicing physician and clinical researcher with an intense passion for phlebology, I suspect that this book will serve as a vein disease primer for both laypersons and primary care physicians alike, and applaud its publication.

Alan H. Kanter, M.D.

Introduction: Who Is This Book For?

Once upon a time, no one thought you could prevent tooth decay...

We all know what a fairy tale that was. Not to say that people never get cavities. Or that there aren't those unfortunate folks who are more susceptible than others to tooth decay. But now we know what we need to do to slow down or prevent the process.

The same might be said about venous disease. Let me explain...

Several years after working in the Intensive Care Unit of a local trauma center, I accepted a position with a physician specializing in venous disease (phlebology). Although I'd suffered from the problem myself, I really knew little about it, making the common erroneous assumption that it was always a purely cosmetic affliction.

I soon learned that, although incurable, the disease is treatable and that there are things you can do to help prevent it. While having treatment, I began incorporating some of the lifestyle changes I'd been learning about. A few months later, I didn't have to hide my legs anymore. But better than that—for the first time since I was a teenager, my legs didn't hurt!

Thus began my crusade. I want to get the word out—there are things you can do to help prevent vein disease and there is hope once you have it. **So if you are one of the millions of people who think there is no way to prevent varicose and spider veins, or think you have to live with them once you've got them, then this book will teach you how to take charge of the health of your legs.**

Another surprise awaited me when I went out on my own to contract with physicians to offer small vein disease treatment to their patients. Suddenly, doctors began to ask me to teach them about venous disease. I wondered why they didn't already know about it. To my amazement, I learned that most medical schools don't include it in their curriculum and that there are many doctors who still believe myths that have long been scientifically disproved.

Why all the confusion? Perhaps, because of the obvious cosmetic aspect, the disease has not been taken seriously. Or maybe it stems from the idea that the disease only affects women (not true) and until recently, most medical research has focused on men. Whatever the reason, the end result has been years of ignorance and myths—both in the lay and medical communities.

This begs the question—if so many health professionals don't know the answers, where does that leave the average person who simply wants to know how to get rid of or prevent the problem?

This book is meant to be a guide for those people and for health care providers who want to give their patients the truth about venous disease—in plain English but with references for more in-depth reading.

It is my hope that this book will dispel the fairy tales about venous disease, once and for all...

Warning - Disclaimer

OVERVIEW

(Read this first for an overall view of the causes and treatments for vein disease. Then read the full text for more details, especially about the parts that may be of special interest to you.)

THE BLOOD CONNECTION

To understand what goes wrong, you need to know that it is "normal" for your blood to leave your heart by one route (arteries) and return by another (veins).

Your heart is the "shipping and receiving" department of your body. It pumps oxygen-enriched blood through the arteries to every organ, exchanging enriched blood for oxygen-depleted blood.

The oxygen-depleted blood returns to the heart through the veins (which are connected to arteries by tiny capillaries) to pick up more oxygen and repeat the cycle.

Assisted by gravity, blood readily flows downward through arteries to your legs. But coming back "uphill" through your veins, your blood needs help from calf and foot muscles, and must be kept from flowing backward by one-way valves in your veins.

ONE-WAY VALVES—THE WEAK LINK

It is these one-way valves—worn, damaged or missing alto-gether—which are the chief cause of vein disease. Valve defects may be the result of pressure increases in deep leg veins from hormonal imbalances, pregnancy, heredity, and many other conditions.

TREATMENTS

Vein disease is incurable but treatable, and usually can be controlled by periodic assessment and occasional maintenance treatment. Being chronic and progressive, vein disease left untreated probably will get worse, and can lead to leg swelling, dark or light pigment changes, hemorrhage, thrombophlebitis, blood clots in deep veins, and leg ulcers.

COMPRESSION STOCKINGS

Graduated compression stockings can help alleviate symptoms, but cannot reverse damage already done. Surgery, sclerotherapy or laser treatment may be necessary to remove diseased and damaged varicose and spider veins.

DOPPLER ULTRASOUND

Before deciding on treatment, your medical history should be reviewed and a thorough leg exam done. Doppler ultrasound, a non-invasive method of detecting changes in blood flow, should be part of this exam.

DUPLEX ULTRASOUND

Duplex ultrasound has replaced invasive x-ray techniques as the prerequisite diagnostic test of choice to pinpoint the invisible diseased veins that flood the surface varicose veins. It therefore serves as a map to the treating physician using either surgery or sclerotherapy to treat varicose veins.

SURGERY

Larger varicose veins are most commonly treated by surgery or sclerotherapy. Surgery, some of which may be done under local anesthesia on an outpatient basis, may include ligation (tying off the vein) and stripping (removing diseased veins). "Office" varicose vein surgery (ambulant phlebectomy) may be done in a doctor's office under local or regional anesthesia.

SCLEROTHERAPY

Recent advances in non-surgical sclerotherapy have produced clinical results on a par with surgery. This treatment—with usually minimal and short-lived pain—has been shown to relieve symptoms in 85% of patients. It consists of a series of tiny injections into diseased veins, followed by leg compression and daily walking.

LASER—THE NEW TECHNOLOGY

The laser offers a great potential for treatment of spider veins, but results will depend on two important factors: (1) Is the laser being used the right one for treating veins? And (2) is the health care provider experienced, well-trained, and proficient? Many questions should be answered before considering treatment. Most vein specialists agree that lasers are not yet cost-effective compared to sclerotherapy for the majority of spider veins in the leg.

BEING AN INFORMED CONSUMER

Before deciding on treatment, the following sections are a "must" read:

✍ Cut to the Chase
✍ Beam Me Up, Scotty!
✍ How to Shop For Treatment
✍ Getting an Audience With the Wizard of Oz

You will learn...

✍ What happens if you don't treat varicose veins?
✍ Is there anything you can do to prevent vein disease?
✍ What can you do to prevent blood clots when you fly?

CHAPTER ONE

B ecause most of this discussion relates to both varicose and spider veins, for the sake of simplicity those terms will be used only if there are differences in the disease process or treatment that need to be pointed out. Instead the terms *venous disease* or *vein disease* will be used as general terms.

WHAT IS VEIN DISEASE?

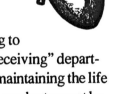

Before we can understand what goes wrong, we need to know what is normal. Let's talk about circulation in general.

Arteries and veins are like the roads leading to and from the heart. The heart is the "shipping and receiving" department of your body. Oxygen and nutrients, vital for maintaining the life of each and every cell, must be distributed. Waste products must be removed.

Like the engine of a delivery truck, the pumping action of the heart continuously drives oxygen-rich blood through the arteries to every organ in the body. A bed of tiny vessels called capillaries connects arteries to veins and allows oxygen to be exchanged for waste products and fluids. Just as the empty truck returns to start the whole process over again, it is the job of veins to carry oxygen-depleted blood back to the heart to pick up more oxygen. This is accomplished by two networks of veins in the legs known as the superficial and the deep venous systems.[7, 8, 18]

The superficial veins are closer to the skin and can be easily seen. Their main job is to help regulate body temperature by dilating or constricting to give off or conserve heat. The superficial veins feed blood to deeper veins via short veins called perforating or communicating veins. The deep veins, with help from muscles in the calf and foot, return blood to the heart. These muscles, called the calf muscle pump or peripheral heart, are the "engine" on the venous end, compressing deep veins, squeezing blood up toward the heart.[9] They play an important role in circulation since the heart does not generate enough pressure to do this job by itself.

Pressure in deep veins is higher than in superficial veins. To keep blood flowing from surface veins to the deep system, leg and arm veins contain a series of one-way valves. They open for uphill flow and close for downhill flow. (see Figures 1 & 2)

Think of blood flow as traffic; valves act like a police officer directing traffic on a congested street. The valve has two flaps that float open during muscle contraction and allow blood to flow toward your heart. During muscle relaxation they close, which prevents blood from flowing backward and pooling in the lower legs.[9,14]

Figure 1

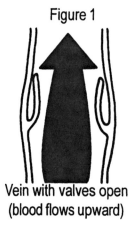

Vein with valves open
(blood flows upward)

Figure 2

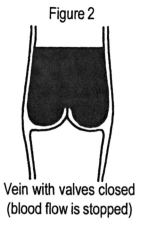

Vein with valves closed
(blood flow is stopped)

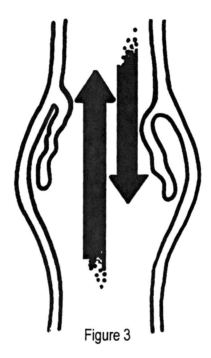

Figure 3

Incompetent valves allow blood to flow upward and backward. When valves become incompetent, blood is allowed to flow in both directions. This leads to sluggish blood flow which can cause swelling and the development of blood clots.

CHAPTER TWO

THE WEAK LINK

The three parts of the venous system of the leg—deep veins, superficial veins, and perforating veins—must work together.
Since they are all connected to one another, it stands to reason that a problem in one leads to a problem in the others.[25]

Unfortunately, the weak link in the whole system is those clever one-way valves. On rare occasions, possibly due to heredity, valves may be absent completely. But more often, veins have widened, creating turbulent blood flow around the valves. They then become thick, just like your finger may form a callus if you play guitar, but, unlike your finger, valves are eventually worn away.[15]

To make things worse, perforating veins (the ones that connect deep and superficial veins) contain lots of valves and are thin-walled, making them more fragile and susceptible to changes in pressure.[10]

Incompetent valves are not able to control blood flow so the calf muscle pump becomes ineffective. (see Figure 3) Venous blood cannot be efficiently returned to the heart because the calf muscle pump is unable to do its job (routing blood back to the deep circulation). When something causes a slowdown or a blockage of venous blood to the heart, it is called venous insufficiency.

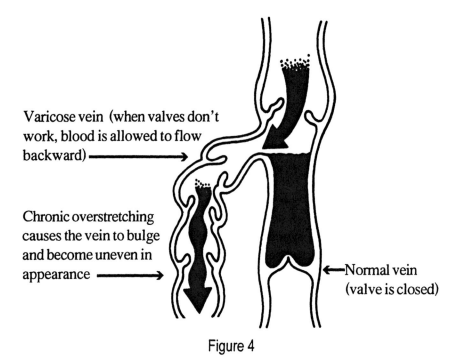

Varicose vein (when valves don't work, blood is allowed to flow backward) ⟶

Chronic overstretching causes the vein to bulge and become uneven in appearance ⟶

⟵ Normal vein (valve is closed)

Figure 4

CHAPTER THREE

A VARICOSE VEIN IS BORN

What goes wrong? Well, for one thing, gravity is against us. Try a little experiment. Sit upright and let your hand hang down at your side. (Be sure there is nothing constricting your arm or wrist.) Notice how the veins in back of your hand pop out? This is due to pressure from gravity. If you raise your hand above the level of your heart, the veins will collapse. This demonstrates the pressure that is always present in the legs when we stand, and how it is relieved when we lie down. And since we don't walk on our hands, we don't get varicose veins in our arms.

Two other important principles apply to fluids; (1) fluids (i.e., blood) always flow downward, like water down a mountain stream, and (2) from points of higher pressure to points of lower pressure.[52] In other words, blood will take the path of least resistance.

Thus, failed venous one-way valves lead to chronic overstretching of veins. Like a balloon blown up too often, veins become stretched out of shape—and a varicose vein is born. (see Figure 4) When we talk about varicose veins, as well as spider veins, we are talking about vessels that no longer function properly. They do not benefit overall circulation, and are generally considered by most experts to be poor candidates for heart surgery by-pass grafts. This is an important distinction, and an often-asked question.

CHAPTER FOUR

SEX, LIES, AND VARICOSE VEINS

Unfortunately, despite ongoing research by physicians specializing in the disease in North America and Europe, ignorance still abounds—both in lay and medical communities—for a couple of reasons. (1), Correct surgical intervention and sclerotherapy are often not taught in medical school or residency programs,[8] and (2), due to its cosmetic nature, venous disease is often ignored—by those suffering from the disease and by physicians who may be uninformed or have little time to deal with problems thought to be more of a nuisance than potentially serious.[63]

CHAPTER FIVE

WHO SAYS REAL MEN DON'T GET VARICOSE VEINS?

Not only is that untrue, but real men also get spider veins. There is no doubt the majority of patients who seek treatment for this disease are women. However, an estimated 80 million adults in the United States alone suffer from leg vein disease,[8] and varicose veins do occur in men. There is an increased incidence with age in both men and women.[12]

According to Wayne M. Marley, MD, past president of the North American Society of Phlebology, the incidence is somewhat less than in women, varying from approximately 10% of men in their 30's up to 40% of men in their 70's. The incidence of spider veins varies and ranges about 20%.

Dr. Marley says most phlebologists find that their practice is predominately female. "In my own practice," he states, "we will see nine women with varicose veins for every man, and probably 99 women with spider veins for every man. I am uncertain as to why there are so few men who seek treatment for symptomatic varicose veins. Certainly men are no more difficult to treat, and can experience the same outcome from a comparable course of therapy.

"Spider veins are probably not as cosmetically embarrassing to men because the hair on men's legs is usually enough to camouflage them. This is, of course, a cultural custom and could vary."

It may also be that men are often hesitant to talk about what is generally thought of as a "woman's" problem.

So how do we get varicose veins?

As we said earlier, heredity can play a role.[62] A very small number of people may be born without valves in their veins. More likely, however, is an inherited tendency for vein wall weakness or valve abnormalities.[17] Standing or sitting occupations are known contributors to vein disease. Also, people with Type A blood have more of a risk.[18]

Anything that increases pressure in deep veins of the legs can lead to vein disease. This can happen when there is a blockage in the system or when pressure in the abdomen is raised. There are a number of common, but preventable causes of increased abdominal pressure which will be discussed later. Rarely, it may be the result of a tumor.[14]

A frequent but overlooked cause of increased abdominal pressure is pregnancy.[14] However, long before the uterus is large enough to cause an increase in pressure—as early as 6 weeks into the pregnancy—venous disease may develop, sometimes even before the first missed menstrual period. **Vein disease is sometimes the first sign of pregnancy!** [16,24,29] Because pregnancy also causes an increase in the actual amount of blood volume,[56] veins are subject to a higher pressure—it's like adding water to an already bulging water balloon.

It is apparent that hormones play a role here, also evidenced by the fact that more women than men suffer from varicose veins. Researchers believe estrogen and progesterone are the culprits, and most likely it is the balance of these two hormones that is important.[16,24,29,56,59] In addition to hormonal changes of pregnancy, the use of oral contraceptives[17] or hormone replacement therapy may promote vein expansion. (Note: We are not advocating that you stop hormone therapy; always talk to your doctor before deciding on any changes in medication.)

While we're talking about hormones, it is worth mentioning that prolonged use of topical steroids also has been shown to cause spider veins.[30]

Pregnancy also increases the risk of thrombophlebitis,[17] which is simply inflammation of a vein associated with a build-up of blood products capable of causing a blockage.[48] (see Figure 5) Besides its potential for destroying valves (leading to varicose vein formation),[14] thrombophlebitis has the potential to lead to pulmonary embolism,[17] which occurs when blood current carries the clot from the vein to a branch of the artery in the lungs, where it causes a potentially life-threatening obstruction.[49]

Trauma may also cause vein disease. Anything that causes damage—from a hit with a tennis ball to a surgical incision—may lead to formation of new blood vessels or cause existing ones to dilate and grow.[31]

Many people will be happy to know that, contrary to popular belief, there is no scientific evidence that crossing your legs causes vein problems.

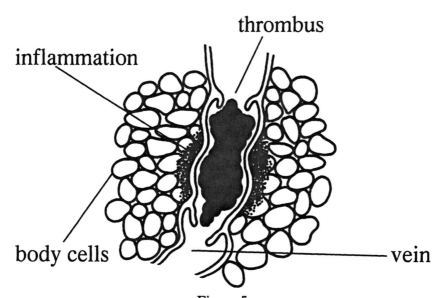

Figure 5
THROMBOPHLEBITIS

CHAPTER SIX

LOOKING FOR VEINS IN ALL THE WRONG PLACES

Diseased veins can show up anywhere on the body. As we mentioned before, trauma can cause vein disease. The most common form of physical damage to the skin is a result of sun exposure. Facial veins, common in both men and women, are often the result of sun damage.

A number of women develop vaginal varicose veins, especially during pregnancy. If veins occurred as a result of pregnancy, they may disappear several weeks after the baby is born. Before treating the veins, a thorough evaluation should be done to determine whether there is an underlying problem in the deep system.[36]

Vein disease, specifically small vein disease, may be an important diagnostic sign of other disorders. It may occur as a result of certain infections or from a collagen vascular disease, such as lupus erythematosis. There are many possible reasons it develops, one being a lack of oxygen to the tissues as a result of the disease process itself.[28]

Varicose veins rarely develop in children but when they do, they are almost always associated with other congenital vascular malformations. [12,57]

A large number of people suffer from leg ulcers, possibly as many as one million in the United States alone.[60] And chronic leg ulcers occur in at least 1% of adults, with venous disease being the most common underlying cause.[66]

Nearly 100,000 Americans are totally disabled by venous ulcers, and the cost for treating ulcers in the United States is estimated to be between $777 million and $1 billion—with an estimated two million work days lost each year![31]

According to Mitchel P. Goldman, MD, author of seven textbooks on the diagnosis and treatment of varicose veins and Assistant Clinical Professor of Dermatology at the University of California, San Diego, "Leg ulcers may be the result of a whole range of problems. They may originate from diseased veins or arteries or arise as a result of an infection or cancer. Although the majority are due to venous disease, proper diagnosis of the cause of the ulcer by a dermatologist or vascular surgeon is the first step in treatment. The underlying cause must be corrected for the ulcer to heal.

"To a degree, the risk factors that predispose one to varicose veins are the same for venous ulcers. The appearance of the ulcer, however, is vein disease at its worst—it signals the end-stage of venous disease. One important note: Poor nutrition, particularly Vitamin C deficiency, plays a significant role in the healing process. Treatment for ulcers should always include a well-balanced diet and your doctor may also prescribe Vitamin C and zinc supplements."

CHAPTER SEVEN

ACHY-BREAKY LEGS

Let's set the record straight once and for all. Varicose and spider veins are not only ugly, they can hurt! Generally, symptoms that occur with larger varicose veins include aches, pains, and night cramps. Swelling, burning, throbbing, a dull aching, (especially after prolonged standing or related to the menstrual cycle), leg cramps, itching, heaviness, and "tired" legs are usually attributed to spider veins. However, symptoms often overlap and are not necessarily related to the size of veins or the extent of disease.[8,12,20,32]

CHAPTER EIGHT

RESTLESS LEGS SYNDROME (RLS)

A common problem (occurring in 5-29% of the American population) which may be associated with iron deficiency, uremia, and diabetes, Restless Legs Syndrome is a chronic condition which runs in families and affects more women than men. Symptoms are made worse by pregnancy.

Characterized by uncomfortable sensations of creeping, tingling, and aching in the legs when sitting or lying down, legs experience a strong urge to move in order to relieve symptoms. Although symptoms may occur any time, many of those with RLS experience them at night, and the discomfort is often severe enough to disturb their sleep (or that of their bed partner).

Most people are unaware that recent research has shown that a great number of those with RLS also suffer from venous disease.

Because of this relationship, RLS sufferers should be evaluated to see if treatment for venous disease may help before being consigned to chronic drug therapy. In a recent study of patients who had both vein disease and RLS, **98%** experienced relief from RLS symptoms after sclerotherapy for their vein disease.[2]

More than half of patients seeking treatment for vein disease do so because of pain and discomfort.[21] It stands to reason then that treating offending veins may eliminate a lot of symptoms. However, it is important to point out that you cannot assume that all leg discomfort comes from veins. There are many other possibilities so a thorough examination with any appropriate tests should always be the first order of business.

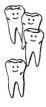

And now, for the good news. Vein disease, although incurable, is treatable, and can usually be maintained by periodic assessment and occasional maintenance treatment,[2] a regimen not unlike regular teeth cleaning.

CHAPTER NINE

TRY A LITTLE TENDERNESS

So what kind of treatment is best?

Let's talk first about the consequences of having no treatment. Once you have venous disease, it will not go away without treatment. There are things you can do to slow down formation of new veins which we will get into a little later, but the old saying, "one thing leads to another" applies. In other words, because of the connection between deep and superficial veins, a problem in one leads to a problem in the other. For many people spider veins are more than a cosmetic nuisance; they may actually be an indication of underlying varicose veins that have not yet been detected.[28]

Venous disease is <u>chronic</u> and <u>progressive</u>, so it makes sense that any diseased vein—varicose or spider—left untreated is probably going to get worse. It's really a matter of degree, with the more serious complications generally occurring with larger varicose veins.

Untreated venous disease can lead to leg swelling, dark or light pigment changes, hemorrhage, thrombophlebitis, blood clots in deep veins, and leg ulcers.[12]

Conservative treatment for venous disease may include graduated compression and walking. Wearing compression stockings—and we are talking specifically about custom-fitted, <u>graduated</u> stockings, not "support" hose generally bought in a department store—can help alleviate symptoms of venous disease by making the calf muscle pump work more efficiently.[37] Unfortunately, although your legs probably will feel lots better while you're wearing them, they can't cure the problem once damage is already done. Without the keeper of blood flow (valves) directing "traffic" between the deep and superficial systems, blood pools and varicose veins form. The only way to get rid of the problem is to close off unhealthy routes by surgery, sclerotherapy, or laser treatment.

Before deciding on what treatment is best, a thorough exam of the legs should be done. The initial exam should include a medical history, and a visual as well as a physical exam of the legs. The Doppler ultrasound, a non-invasive method for detecting changes in blood flow, should be part of this exam.[3,26,33,65] There are other tests that may be performed depending on the findings so far. It is important to determine if there is a problem in the arteries and to rule out the possibility of a clot in the deep veins before treatment.

A Duplex scanner (also called Duplex imaging) is an ultrasound machine that uses an imaging probe (kind of like watching your veins on a TV screen) to visualize superficial and deep blood vessels, as well as to determine direction of blood flow.[34] Not everyone needs to be examined with the Duplex scanner, but for those contemplating treatment for varicose (versus spider) veins, it is an important tool. Because the three components of the venous system are all connected—superficial veins, perforating veins, and deep veins—it is important to determine where the problem originates before treating it. If there is a problem in the deep system but only superficial varicose veins are treated, treatment may not be effective. It would be like trying to plug a hole in a fire hose by blocking the nozzle—the water will still leak out the hole.

Even if you are contemplating surgery for your varicose veins, the Duplex scanner can target problem veins, assisting the surgeon in localizing and treating those areas.[23] If sclerotherapy is chosen, the Duplex Scanner is able to pinpoint abnormalities in the connection between arterial and venous systems[68] enabling a more effective and safer treatment.[21] With the use of the scanner, underlying problem veins that previously were accessible only through surgery can be eliminated[61] with the advantage of real-time feedback showing that the targeted vessels are the ones actually treated.

And lastly, the scanner is a great tool as a follow-up to treatment to evaluate its effectiveness[34] as well as helping in early detection of recurrences. One important note: Duplex scanning should be done by qualified physicians or technicians with specialized training in vascular screening.

CHAPTER TEN

CUT TO THE CHASE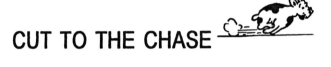

Now that you know what to expect from the exam, it's time to get down to brass tacks. What are the treatment options?

With both varicose and spider veins, treatment may be a combination of options. Let's talk first about larger varicose veins.

The two most commonly used methods are surgery and sclerotherapy. Used properly, they both have a role in controlling venous disease. Ligation (tying off the vein) and stripping (removing diseased veins through small incisions using a special tool) have been used for many years. Modifications have been made over the years aimed at preserving healthy veins while pinpointing more precisely those that are diseased. Depending on the type of surgical procedure used, some can be done under local anesthesia on an outpatient basis.[50]

Some of potential surgical complications include hemorrhage, hematoma (a localized collection of blood), and nerve damage,[5] as well as risks from anesthesia.

Ambulant phlebectomy originated in Europe and has gained popularity in the United States in the last seven or eight years. It may be used alone or in conjunction with other treatments. As the name implies, this is done in the doctor's office and usually under local or regional anesthesia. It is effective on the size veins normally considered for "stripping" and has the presumed advantage of achieving the same long-term results as surgery with a more convenient, less expensive procedure. Complications are generally less frequent and milder than with traditional vein stripping.[5]

Whatever surgical method is used, the preoperative history and exam should be thorough, and veins to be removed should be marked carefully prior to surgery after identification by Duplex ultrasound.[5,50]

Sclerotherapy, a series of tiny injections into diseased veins causing them to sclerose or harden, is a non-surgical procedure that's also been around for decades. Earlier treatment efforts often led to poor results. In spite of the introduction of safer medications in the 1940s and the addition of compression after treatment in the 1960s (considered to be one of the most important advances in sclerotherapy),[8,37] many people are still unaware that clinical results equal to surgical procedures are now reported.[8,64] In addition, research also has shown that sclerotherapy relieves symptoms in 85% of patients.[21]

Since the 1960's, sclerotherapy has been fully accepted by the medical community in Europe and exists as a separate specialty. However, even today, many American physicians are unclear about the treatment, harboring **erroneous** perceptions that sclerotherapy destroys veins indiscriminately, has a high risk for blood clots and allergic reactions, and won't produce much improvement—just to name a few. A recent survey found that 82% of gynecologists surveyed did not have enough knowledge to advise patients who requested information on the treatment of varicose veins and spider veins.[12]

How does sclerotherapy work?

After diseased veins are injected, medication causes them to collapse. Application of compression right after treatment helps seal veins, and along with daily walks, helps reroute blood away from surface vessels and into deep veins. Eventually, what was a hollow tube becomes a solid thread of scar tissue. A note about compression: Depending on the severity of the disease, other forms of compression may be used, such as tapes or bandages. Although expensive, graduated compression hose are the "Cadillac" of compression and if properly cared for should last at least 4 to 6 months. So do your legs a favor and wear them if they are prescribed. They are far superior to anything else and may even help make your treatments more effective.

Walking, along with the proper compression, is a vital part of the treatment—as much as the injections themselves. It helps minimize potential risks of sclerotherapy and is so important that this procedure should not be used on people who are unable to walk[51] or will not commit to a daily walking program.

Except with the most minor spider veins, more than one treatment is necessary, along with a certain amount of follow-up care.

As a result of treatment—actually, it is the goal of treatment—diseased veins become sealed off from the rest of the circulation and blood inside them gets "trapped." Depending on the size of the vein, these pockets of trapped blood sometimes become tender and may even feel lumpy. They should be removed in subsequent visits.[45,47] This is a *normal* result of treatment but it's important to understand that *your legs will look worse before they look better.* Removal of trapped blood, along with adequate compression and daily walking, help the vein to seal shut and thus, speed up the healing process. (Without the walking and compression, the vein may re-open.)

Until complete closure of the vein has occurred, small amounts of blood may leak back into it, requiring further treatment of trapped blood. This part of the treatment process should not be neglected. Left untreated, trapped blood can take many months to be reabsorbed by the body. Meanwhile, iron in blood may react with skin to leave a persistant "stain" (resembling a shadow of the vein).[20]

Some patients with long-standing varicose veins may already have this staining simply from so much blood being in close contact with skin over time. Unfortunately, this will not resolve even when veins are treated[22] and emphasizes the need for those who have had sclerotherapy to keep any follow-up appointments, even after all treatment is completed.

In spite of that, a small percentage of people may be left with some amount of staining, from the iron in blood mentioned before, or possibly due to inflammation that occurs during normal treatment, which may stimulate excessive deposit of skin pigment.[22] However, although skin discoloration after treatment is a relatively common occurrence after sclerotherapy, and may take up to a year or two to resolve, the percentage of people left with a permanent stain is very small.[44]

As treated larger varicose veins become sealed, you may feel a firm cord along the path of the vein.[39] This is normal, and as the cord is slowly reabsorbed by the body, you may experience sensations of pulling, like a rubber band stretching.

Prior to starting sclerotherapy treatment, as with surgery, you should be given an informed consent to read and sign. By being aware of potential complications, you give yourself the opportunity to play a more active role in your treatment. Some risks include hyperpigmentation (the excessive deposit of skin pigment mentioned previously) which is usually temporary, but may in rare cases be permanent. Except in the case of hypertonic saline, as with any medication, an allergic reaction can occur, which may be mild or life-threatening. However, because hypertonic saline is very painful, sometimes anesthetics are added to the solution which have the potential to cause an allergic reaction. It should be pointed out that localized itching and wheals (raised patches of skin) occur after injection of all sclerotherapy medications, but usually last only for a short time (approximately 30 minutes).[45]

Because very tiny needles are used for this procedure, pain is minimal and usually short-lived. The medication used can make a difference, however; for example, hypertonic saline is notorious for causing pain and cramping.[45] Temporary swelling may occur, usually in the ankle area if it has been treated.

Sometimes the body's response to shutting down veins is to create new ones. They are usually very fine and red in color and are known as "matting." Although rarely a permanent problem, matting may take 3 to 12 months to resolve.[45] Laser or expert sclerotherapy treatment may be effective in eliminating matting that persists beyond a reasonable time period.

Due to the fact that all sclerotherapy medications act by irritating the blood vessel, even with expert technique, skin ulceration and underlying tissue damage is possible. Generally fairly small, the ulcer may take 4-6 weeks to heal and may leave a small scar.[45]

Thrombophlebitis, deep vein thrombosis, arterial injections, and nerve damage are relatively rare complications.[44] It is very important to give a complete medical history so other potential risks may be assessed.

Note: People often worry that getting rid of so many veins will hurt their circulation. This is not true; there are hundreds of veins in your legs and treatment is only applied to the diseased veins.

Who Should Not Have Treatment?

Anyone who is bedridden or unable to walk should not have sclerotherapy. Pregnant women should also avoid it. It is a good idea to wait about 6 weeks after childbirth before seeking vein treatment (including surgical treatment) because often some diseased veins may disappear. Some physicians will treat breastfeeding women as long as they do not breastfeed for 24 hours after treatment.

If you are contemplating surgery other than vein stripping, wait for an okay from your doctor after surgery before having sclerotherapy treatment. If you have a history of thrombophlebitis or deep vein thrombosis you should be tested first to see if you are a candidate for treatment. If you are taking Antabuse, certain sclerotherapy medications must be avoided so others would have to be substituted. If you have had an allergic reaction to a medication used in sclerotherapy, another one may be used. Once again, the medical history you give prior to the start of treatment is vital.

CHAPTER ELEVEN

BEAM ME UP, SCOTTY!

Light Amplification by Stimulated Emission of Radiation — LASER — the very name evokes images of space-age magical treatment. But before you succumb to this seductive technology, bear in mind that results will depend on two important factors: (1) Is the laser being used the right one for treating veins, and (2) Is the health care provider well-trained?

No matter what its potential, a piece of equipment is only as good as the expertise behind it. Don't be seduced by the mere fact that the laser is available. Laser is being used in many areas of medicine with wonderful results, but the technology is still fairly new. The consumer should be aware that, as of this writing, no national standards exist for laser training.

A little anecdote will demonstrate. Back in the 1950's when X-ray was not widely understood, a well-known shoe store thought it would be a great idea if people could actually "see" how well their shoes fit when they tried them on. They had x-ray tubes installed in the floor, the customer would step on a little box and they could see their bones illuminated, proving what a great fit the shoes were.

It was a great sales gimmick -- until the sales people started getting skin cancers on their faces, developed cataracts, and thyroid problems.

The point being made is, that in well-trained hands in a safe environment, X-ray was and continues to be a vital tool. The same can be said for laser.

(Note: These same questions generally apply to seeking laser treatment for other things, too. However, the following applies specifically to vein disease.)

How Does It Work?

Light is made up of photons. Originally defined by Einstein, a photon is simply a packet of radiated energy. For example, light from a light bulb is a stream of photons. The photons have electromagnetic properties which are useful because they are predictable and consistent.

Light travels in waves with peaks and valleys. The distance between two "peaks" determines the wave length. Some wave lengths have the ability to be "selectively absorbed" by different materials. This enables the use of energy that is minor enough to pass through the skin without significant damage to that tissue, while creating enough energy to close the vessel. Like light shining through a window, this specific light energy is passed through skin where it causes the vein to rapidly become heated. The vein "burns" closed.

If you've ever burned a hole in a piece of paper using a magnifying glass and sunlight, it's easy to understand that light can burn. The trick is to "control" the burn. Without this control, damage to other tissues will occur. By utilizing the unique characteristics of laser light to cause an exact effect, the burn can be controlled. The "burn" is actually photocautery, or the burning of the vein by laser light.

Other important factors are the amount of time light is in contact with the skin (which may be thought of as the "dose" of light used), as well as the wattage (which may be thought of as the quantity).

Different wave lengths are chosen to do different tasks. What this really means is that you cannot assume that just because laser is used, it will do a good job. Lasers are as specific as tools in a tool box. Would it make sense to use a screw driver to hammer a nail when you have a hammer available? Although most lasers would be capable of getting rid of spider veins, one of the biggest problems in using the wrong laser is destruction of healthy tissue along with diseased veins—like shooting a rabbit with a cannon.

Is It Safe?

If the answer to questions (1) and (2) in the first paragraph of this section are yes, then the answer to this question is yes. Low doses of energy are used, which minimizes risk of significant injury to the skin. Because tiny blood vessels being treated are below the surface of the skin, bleeding is not a problem. However, it should be noted that protective eyewear should be worn by everyone in the room any time laser is being used.

Does It Always Work?

The success of laser treatment is very dependent on the expertise of the practitioner. Laser is most effective on the smallest spider veins so it is important to treat larger "feeder vessels" by sclerotherapy prior to treatment with laser.

Other factors, such as dry, flaky skin and the presence of lotion on skin can adversely affect treatment and should be taken into account by the practitioner. In general, lesions may need up to three treatments to be eliminated, and a small percentage of patients may have poor results.

How Can You Be Sure You Are Getting The Best Treatment?

This type of treatment should not cause bruising, severe pain, or major changes in the skin, or require major lifestyle alterations during the healing phase, and there should be visible change after each treatment. Bruising or burns beyond simple welting are signs of the use of an incorrect energy pattern. Both of these complications can cause permanent marks on the skin.

The success of laser treatment, as is often the case with other medical procedures, is dependent on the proficiency of the therapist. How many times a day, on average, does the practitioner perform this treatment? Studies have shown that successful repetition of a procedure is generally an indication of a good success rate.

Is It Painful?

The sensation is generally described as warm and sharp, like the snap of a rubber band against the skin. Ice may be used to cool the areas being treated and over-the-counter analgesics may be taken, but anesthetics are not necessary.

Is It Permanent?

While it may take two or three treatments to close the vessel, if the treatment is done efficiently and on veins of the appropriate size (tiny), the vessels are not liable to reopen. However, as with other therapies, this is not a cure for vein disease and will require occasional maintenance. Remember that sclerotherapy should generally be done first to treat the "feeder veins" before laser is used on the smaller vessels.

How Many Visits Will It Take?

The number of visits varies with the individual's perception of "being done," the number of veins needing treatment, and the physical health of the patient. An individual assessment must be done to determine the amount of therapy needed; five hours of treatment is a reasonable average.

How Long Does It Take To Heal?

This varies greatly from patient to patient. Most patients will develop a scab that looks like a cat scratch which may resolve in a few days, but may take up to six weeks. The average healing time is two weeks, but elderly patients and those in poor health will have much longer healing periods. To avoid scarring, these areas should not be scratched or picked at.

Is There Anyone Who Should Not Have Treatment With Laser?

People in poor health will not respond well. As with other therapies, pregnant women should wait to allow vein disease to subside after childbirth before having treatment. People with Lupus may have a negative effect from the intense light of the laser. Darker skinned patients are at higher risk of developing loss of pigment and should receive treatment by practitioners who have had experience working with various skin tones. And lastly, patients with unrealistic expectations of the treatment or the results should not have treatment.

CHAPTER TWELVE

HOW TO SHOP FOR TREATMENT

In shopping for health care, as in anything else, it pays to become an informed consumer. Get information over the phone, schedule a consultation and if necessary, get a second opinion. Make sure you understand all your options, as well as the risks before you have any procedure done.

Questions To Ask

- Has the FDA approved the treatment or medication being used? (If covered by their malpractice insurance, some health care providers use non-FDA approved medications for sclerotherapy which may be very effective and safe. However, you still have the right to know.)
- What kind of training did you receive in preparation for offering this treatment? (Has the course been accredited through the American Medical Association for category 1 continuing medical education credits or the American Nurses' Association for continuing education credits,[55] or has it been approved by a state board of nursing?)
- How many of these procedures have you done?
- How often do you see complications with this procedure?
- What do you do to stay current in your field? (professional memberships, continuing education, etc.)

In addition, you can call your State Medical Board or Board of Registered Nursing for information about any complaints.

CHAPTER THIRTEEN

GETTING AN AUDIENCE WITH THE WIZARD OF OZ

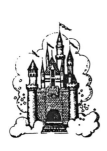

It's fair to say that Dorothy probably had less trouble getting an audience with Oz than it may be to get price information over the phone. Fair enough. You would never expect a body repair shop to give you an estimate on repairing your car over the phone or a heart surgeon to give you an estimate on surgery without doing an exam. Having your veins treated may not be as critical as cardiac surgery but still deserves your efforts to find the right practitioner. Your family physician or a happy patient may be able to refer you to someone but you should invest the time to meet the practitioner for consultation and decide based on personal impression and the answers to your questions. If you do "shop around," <u>make sure you're comparing apples with apples.</u>

Money should not be the only consideration—experience and level of expertise as well as successful results are equally (if not more) important. However, whether treatment is affordable is a key question and you have the right to know exactly what costs are involved. Here are some questions to ask:

- How much is the consultation and is it applied to the cost of treatment?

- What exactly does the consultation consist of? What tests, if any, will cost extra?
- In the case of sclerotherapy and laser treatment - How much does a treatment cost and what does it consist of? For example, with sclerotherapy, it may take multiple treatments of hundreds of injections to clear up veins. If one treatment costs $125 and consists of ten injections (which can be done in about 2 minutes) while another costs $200 but will provide as many injections as can be done in 15 minutes, it doesn't take long to figure that the $200 treatment is a better deal.
- Do you give a written cost estimate? This should list the cost of each treatment as well as an estimate for the number of treatments needed to clear up the problem. Left open-ended, you could end up paying a lot of money for very little work and be in treatment for months. If you know how much a treatment costs but you don't know how many treatments are needed, how can you possibly figure out the cost? Make sure the written estimate also covers the cost of any compression needed and follow-up appointments.
- Do you need pre-authorization, which means your insurance has agreed to pay for all or part of your treatment? While it is rarely needed for out-patient non-surgical sclerotherapy, it is required for in-patient procedures and most surgery.
- Does the health care provider accept assignment? If the health care provider accepts assignment, it means it is willing to settle for the amount your insurance pays for treatment. Most health care providers will not accept assignment because it usually amounts to far less than the actual bill. If assignment is not accepted, you will be responsible for whatever your insurance does not pay. If you belong to an HMO, check to see if the health care provider is authorized to be paid for performing the treatment under your plan (this usually is not covered). If so, it must be pre-approved by the HMO before you begin treatment. Otherwise, it will not pay.
- If you don't have insurance coverage, is it possible to make payments? Most health care providers will accept credit cards, although only a few may have payment plans.

CHAPTER FOURTEEN

AN OUNCE OF PREVENTION IS WORTH A POUND OF CURE

Although vein disease is a chronic and progressive condition, you can do some things to help slow down development of the problem. For those who are having treatment for vein disease, applying these same preventive measures ensures you will get the most out of the treatment.

Anyone who is about to undergo surgery or who is bedridden or pregnant, should ask their doctor if they should be fitted with a graduated support stocking because these groups are all at higher risk for deep vein thrombosis (blood clots).[12]

Earlier we noted that vein disease may be the first sign of pregnancy. In addition to the prevention of blood clots, many uncomfortable symptoms which occur in the legs during pregnancy may be relieved by the use of compression stockings.[58] These come in maternity sizes, must be made to measure, and may be covered by insurance.

Let's talk a little more about graduated compression hose. First of all, a graduated stocking is tightest at the ankle, gradually becoming looser (but not loose) as it goes up. This helps reduce swelling and augments the calf muscle pump, improving blood flow through the deep veins.[37]

Regular support hose feel good because they support the muscles. The larger the leg, the better they will feel but they don't help the efficiency of the calf muscle pump.

Unfortunately, non-graduated compression may actually cause more harm than good by creating a tourniquet effect. This applies to most "support" hose usually sold in department stores as well as any kind of bandage applied unevenly to the legs.

The manufacturing process is what sets graduated compression hose apart from other stockings which begin as "tube socks" that are then shaped with heat around a metal leg form. Graduated compression hose are knit into the proper anatomical leg shape from the start, a more expensive method that enables the manufacturer to guarantee that the compression is both correct and graduated.

Note: Height and weight measurements will not provide the kind of fit (or a guarantee of a certain amount of compression) that ankle, calf, and thigh measurements will. For example, if you took five women who are 5 ft. 7 in. - 5 ft. 10 in. tall and weigh between 140-160 lbs. and measured the ankle, calf, and thigh of each, you might find ankle circumference differences of 2-3 inches and calf circumference differences of 3-5 inches. It is easy to see then why the same size stocking will not deliver the same amount of graduated compression.

There are several degrees of compression, measured in millimeters of mercury (mm Hg). It takes as little as 18 mm Hg of ankle pressure to augment the calf muscle pump. The stockings are worn for a variety of conditions, ranging from light swelling or fatigue to prevention of varicose veins during pregnancy to more serious vein disease. The amount of compression depends on why stockings are being worn, and those with higher compression may require a prescription. (See appendix for guide to ordering compression and prescription form.)

If high compression is needed and stockings are difficult to apply, two lower compression stockings can be worn one over the other. Also, as mentioned before, adequate compression is an important part of sclerotherapy treatment and helps minimize potential risks of treatment.[39] Note: If legs are swollen, they should be elevated for five or ten minutes above the level of the heart before applying stockings.

For those at risk for vein disease who sit or stand for prolonged periods (as well as during pregnancy), wearing graduated compression can help slow down formation of diseased veins. Not only that, but many uncomfortable symptoms of fatigue and heaviness may be avoided.

But don't despair! In recent years graduated compression hose have come a long way—with new fabrics and colors, these stockings have become much more stylish. There's something for everyone— knee highs and men's socks that are also great under jeans and casual pants, sexy thigh-highs with a lacy tops, sheer pantyhose, soft, ribbed-knit tights—just to name a few. And, although there are still some available in that horrible color we all associate with "therapeutic" hose, most are also available in yummy colors. In short, there is no longer any reason to give up style in order to wear graduated compression. (A comparison of graduated support hose can be found in the appendix.)

Many are now available online and at prices competitive with name brand support hose. For example, check out Ames Walker Support Hosiery at www.supporthosiery.com

CHAPTER FIFTEEN

I'M GONNA WALK THOSE VEINS RIGHT OUT OF MY LEGS

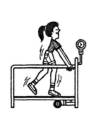 **Probably the single most important thing you can do to help slow down the progression of venous disease is to walk regularly.**

Experts believe that walking can help prevent vein disease. In addition, it has other important health benefits. Recent research has shown that men as well as women can experience osteoporosis, which leads to loss of bone density and weaker bones with a higher risk for fractures. Drugs may be used to combat the problem, but regular weight-bearing exercise may help prevent it from occurring in the first place. This is simply because bone responds to muscle action by becoming stronger (and when there is no muscle action, bone becomes weaker).

Some patients discover their restless legs symptoms diminish with regular walking. It may be coincidental, but there is no dispute that regular walking helps prevent heart disease, relieves stress and is a great way to get in shape! Because it is inexpensive, convenient, requires no special equipment or training, and has a low risk of injury, it is an easy way to add the exercise component to a change in diet that is essential to weight control.

Prevention of vein disease, osteoporosis, heart disease and obesity—if that isn't enough, the sense of well-being that comes with a regular exercise program will inspire you to make a life long commitment to walking.

If you are having sclerotherapy on your legs, walking is an important part of the treatment, helping to minimize potential risks by diluting the medication, keeping blood flow from becoming stagnant, and decreasing the risk of serious clots. It is so important that if you cannot walk, you should not have treatment.[47]

Because of the squeezing action of muscles in the leg and calf, walking helps keep pressure from surface vessels low,[52] rerouting blood to deep vessels where it belongs.

Avoid standing or sitting for prolonged periods. If it cannot be avoided, gently rock from the tips of your toes to your heels (this can be done while sitting) or walk for five minutes every hour. If prolonged sitting or standing is part of your normal day, or if you are doing prolonged traveling (including flying), wear your compression hose.

Exercises that cause veins to dilate may increase the risk of venous disease. These include high impact aerobics such as running and jogging, and weight lifting using heavy weights that cause abdominal straining.[14,47] If you are having sclerotherapy treatment, these things must be avoided during, and for a few weeks after, treatment. (Weight lifting using lighter weights for many repetitions for toning is OK.)

CHAPTER SIXTEEN

DANGER IN THE SKIES

It has long been known that people who sit for prolonged periods of time without moving are at risk for the development of blood clots. A recent study published in 1996 takes this information a step further and points out specific risks related to air travel.[68] They are:

- low humidity in the cabin
- lowered oxygen levels
- fluid loss as a result of drinking alcoholic beverages
- insufficient fluid intake (non-alcoholic)
- smoking
- sitting with legs in a dependent position for lengthy periods

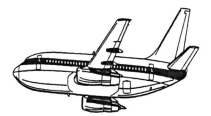

All these can lead to dehydration, stagnant blood flow, and an increase in the ability of the blood to coagulate. People with an added risk are those who:

- have a history of blood clots
- have a chronic disease or cancer
- are on hormone therapy
- have had a recent injury to a lower limb
- have had recent surgery or femoral catheterization

LIFESAVING TIPS FOR PREVENTING BLOOD CLOTS WHEN YOU FLY

- Drink at least 1 liter (almost a quart) of non-alcoholic (and caffeine-free) fluid for every five hours of flight.

- Get up and walk in the aisles for 5 minutes every hour and/or move your legs and feet and take deep breaths every hour. (see Figure 6)

- Keep alcoholic beverages to a minimum.

- After injury or surgery, it may be advisable to wait 6 weeks before air travel. Check with your doctor.

- Some people with added risk factors may benefit by wearing graduated compression hose during the flight. Check with your doctor to see if you are a candidate.

- People who have had previous blood clots, recent surgery, or who have a chronic disease or malignancy should ask their doctor to prescribe low-dose blood-thinning medication.

Simple Exercises to Encourage Venous Blood Flow

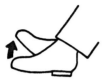

Move your foot up and down

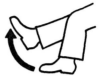

Extend your lower legs

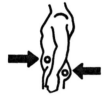

Contract the muscles in your
abdomen and buttocks

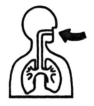

Breathe deeply

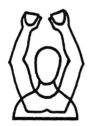

Stretch your arms

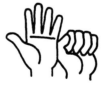

Close and open your hands

Figure 6

TOP TIPS FOR PREVENTING VARICOSE VEINS

Things to do:

- After checking with your doctor, start a walking program
- If you wear support hose, choose graduated compression
- Eat a high fiber diet - *Although unproven, the amount of fiber in the diet, along with other dietary factors, may help prevent formation of vein disease. Some research has found the incidence of vein disease to be related to amount of fiber eaten, with those eating unprocessed high-fiber food free of varicose veins.* [14]
- Control your weight [14]
- While in sclerotherapy treatment, wear compression hose to sleep, if prescribed
- Wear compression hose when flying [27] or on long car trips; get up and walk around every two hours
- Have legs reassessed periodically - *Besides the fact that vein disease is a chronic condition often requiring periodic maintenance treatment, research suggests spider veins may be associated with underlying venous disease.* [23,28]

> Don't stand if you can sit. Don't sit if you can lie down, and if you lie down, elevate your legs above the level of your heart. ♥

Things to avoid:

- Alcohol,[14] hot showers, Jacuzzis and hot tubs[47] - *All cause the veins to dilate.*
- Smoking
- Excessive sun exposure[31] - *Causes trauma to the skin leading to spider vein formation.*
- Constrictive clothing such as girdles[14] - *Causes increased abdominal pressure leading to increased pressure in the legs.*
- Excessively high heels - *May prevent the calf muscle pump from being activated.* [27]
- Non-graduated "support" hose - *Wear only graduated support.* [41]

THE CARE AND FEEDING OF GRADUATED COMPRESSION HOSE

- Sweat and oils from skin and lotion are hard on some stockings so they should be washed frequently. (Most stockings should not come in contact with ointments or creams either.) Use only a mild detergent, such as Ivory Liquid or Dreft and avoid Woolite and bleaches as they may destroy some of the fabrics. Especially in the case of heavier compression stockings, it is a good idea to have two pairs so they can be washed daily. Each manufacturer has specific washing and drying instructions that are important to follow for prolonging the life of the hose as well as complying with warranty requirements.

- Be careful of long fingernails and jewelry. Wear rubber gloves to put on or take off hose to help prevent snagging and make them easier to apply. Stockings will go on easier if you apply a little talcum powder to your legs first.

- When applying stockings be sure not to pull them from the top band up your leg—this will stretch the top half of the stocking and will cause them to "creep down" your leg throughout the day. Spread the fabric evenly along the entire leg.

- Keep toenails trimmed and remove rough skin from feet. Wear shoes that will not snag or wear a hole in the stocking.

- Don't walk around the house in your stockings—wear shoes or slippers.

- If you get a hole in your stocking, don't use nail polish on it—it may dissolve the fabric. You may be able to temporarily prolong the life of the stocking by carefully stitching up the hole.

- Avoid "toe blowout" by grabbing the toe of the hose after you have them on and giving it a gentle tug.

REFERENCES

1. Leg Veins. Harvard Women's Health Watch 1994;Feb:4-5.
2. Kanter AH. The effect of sclerotherapy on restless legs syndrome. Dermatol Surg 1995;21:328-32.
3. Weiss RA and Weiss MA. Doppler ultrasound findings in reticular veins of the thigh subdermic lateral venous system and implications for sclerotherapy. J Dermatol Surg Oncol 1993;19:947-51.
4. Neumann HAM. Ambulant minisurgical phlebectomy. J Dermatol Surg Oncol 1992;18:53-4.
5. Ricci S and Georgiev M. Office varicose veins surgery under local anesthesia. J Dermatol Surg Oncol 1992;18:55-8.
6. Goldman MP. Compression in the treatment of leg telangiectasia: theoretical considerations. J Dermatol Surg Oncol 1989;15:184-8.
7. Cahall E, Spence R. Nursing management of venous ulceration. J Vasc Nurs 1994;June:48-56.
8. Goldman MP. Sclerotherapy: treatment of varicose and telangiectatic leg veins. St. Louis:Mosby-Year Book Inc 1995:ix, 1-8.
9. Ibid. 16-20.
10. Ibid. 28-30.
11. Ibid. 42-3.
12. Ibid. 48-72.
13. Ibid. 69-71.
14. Ibid. 89-96.
15. Ibid. 96-103.
16. Ibid. 103-8.
17. Ibid. 107-8.
18. Ibid. 109-10.
19. Shields JL, Jansen GT. Therapy for superficial telangiectasias of the lower extremities. J Dermatol Surg Oncol 1982;Oct:857-60.
20. Banning GL. Varicose veins and intracutaneous telangiectasia: combined treatment in 1,500 cases. South Med J 1987;Sept:1105-10.
21. Goldman MP. Sclerotherapy treatment for varicose and telangiectatic veins in the United States: past, present and future. J Dermatol Surg Oncol 1990;Jul:606-7.
22. Georgiev M. Postsclerotherapy hyperpigmentation: a one-year follow-up. J Dermatol Surg Oncol 1990;Jul:608-10.
23. Thibault P, et al. Cosmetic leg veins: evaluation using duplex venous imaging. J Dermatol Surg Oncol 1990;Jul:612-18.
24. Sadick NS, Niedt GW. A study of estrogen and progesterone receptors in spider telangiectasias of the lower extremities. J Dermatol Surg Oncol 1990;Jul:620-23.

25. Goldman MP. Sclerotherapy: treatment of varicose and telangiectatic leg veins. St. Louis:Mosby-Year Book Inc 1995:85-94.

26. Hagood CO Jr, Mozersky DJ, Tumblin RN. Practical office techniques for physiologic vascular testing. South Med J 1975;Jan:17-21.

27. Weihermuller M, ed. Practical ambulant phlebology. Garching near Munich: Schorsch-Druck 1991:7-83.

28. Goldman MP. Sclerotherapy: treatment of varicose and telangiectatic leg veins. St. Louis:Mosby-Year Book Inc 1995:130-2.

29. Ibid. 133-4.

30. Ibid. 134-5.

31. Ibid. 135-7.

32. Ibid. 145.

33. Ibid. 155-66.

34. Ibid. 166-70.

35. Ibid. 174-80.

36. Ibid. 193-4.

37. Ibid. 200-6.

38. Ibid. 206.

39. Ibid. 219-21.

40. Ibid. 222-3.

41. Ibid. 223-4.

42. Ibid. 244-6.

43. Ibid. 250-1.

44. Ibid. 280.

45. Ibid. 287-337.

46. Ibid. 322-4.

47. Ibid. 368-9.

48. Friel JP ed. Dorland's illustrated medical dictionary. USA:WB Saunders Co 1974:1606-7.

49. Ibid. 506.

50. Goldman MP. Sclerotherapy: treatment of varicose and telangiectatic leg veins. St. Louis:Mosby-Year Book Inc 1995:394-5.

51. Stemmer R. Sclerotherapy of varicose veins. St Gallen Switzerland:Ganzoni & Cie AG 1990:35.

52. Ibid. 10.

53. Goldman MP. Sclerotherapy: treatment of varicose and telangiectatic leg veins. St. Louis:Mosby-Year Book Inc 1995:144.

54. Goldman MP, Fitzpatrick RE. Cutaneous laser surgery. St. Louis Mosby-Year Book Inc 1994:2.

55. Ibid. 261-2.

56. Skudder PA, Farrington DT. Venous conditions associated with pregnancy. Seminars in Dermatol 1993;12:72-7.

57. Sadick NS. Predisposing factors of varicose and telangiectatic leg veins. J

Dermatol Surg Oncol 1992;18:883-6.

58. Nilsson L, Austrell C, Norgren L. Venous function during late pregnancy, the effect of elastic compression hosiery. Vasa Band 21 1992:203-5.

59. Dindelli M, Parazzine F, Bassellini A. Rabaiotti E, Corsi G, Ferrari A. Risk factors for varicose vein disease before and during pregnancy. J Vasc Diseases 1993;May:361-7.

60. Coon, WW, Willis PW III, Keller JB. Venous thromboembolism and other venous disease in the Tecumseh Community Health Study. Circulation 1973;48:839.

61. Kanter A, Gardner M, Isaacs M. Identification of arteriovenous anastamosis by duplex ultrasound: implications for the treatment of varicose veins. Dermatol Surg 1995;21:—.

62. Service de Cardiologie. Importance of the familial factor in varicose disease: clinical study of 134 families. Dermatol Surg Oncol 1994;20(5):318-26.

63. Evans CJ, et al. Epidemiology of varicose veins: a review. Int Angiol 1994;13(3)263-70.

64. Sugano NIT. Study on thrombus formation and the course of healing after sclerotherapy for varicose veins of the leg [preliminary report]. Int J Cardiol 1994;47(1 Suppl):S65-9.

65. Bradbury AW, et al. Recurrent varicose veins: assessment of the saphenofemoral junction. Br J Surg1994;8(3):373-5.

66. Wipke-Tevis DD, Stotts NA. Nutritional risk, status, and intake of individuals with venous ulcers: a pilot study. J Vasc Nurs 1996;June:27-33.

67. Eklof B, Kistner RL, Masuda EM, Sonntag BV, Wong HP. Venous thromboembolism in association with prolonged air travel. Dermatol Surg 1996; 22:637-641.

68 Kanter A. Thibault PK, Saphenofemoral incompetence treated by ulstrsound-guided sclerotherapy. Dermatol Surg 1996:648-52.

For More on Laser ...

Lasers in America 1950-1970; Joan Lisa Bromberg; the MIT Press, 1991

"Microwave Spectoscopy"; C.H. Townes; Amercian Scientist 40(1952), 270-290

"The Invention of LASER and MASER"; (n.d.) C.H. Townes Papers, File "MASER-LASER History": C.H. Townes, interview by W.V. Smith, June 1979, Niels Bohr Library, American Institute of Physics

"Amplification of Microwave Radiation by Substances not in Thermal

Equilibrium"; J. Weber, Transaction of the IRE Professional Group on Electron Devises PGED-3; June 1953, 1-4

"A History of Engineering and Science in the Bell System: Service in War and Peace" (1925-1975); (Bell Laboratories, 1978) p. 356

"Gaseous Optical MASERS"; A. Javan, in Laser Applications; Applied Optics; Supplement 1. (1962) p. 35

Mitchell P. Goldman and Richard E. Fitzpatrick, Cutaneous Laser Surgery (St. Louis: Mosby - Year Book, Inc., 1994)

Appendices

COMPARISON OF GRADUATED COMPRESSION HOSE

According to a survey by the National Association of Hosiery Manufacturers, the average woman buys 10-18 pairs of hose a year, wearing each pair of pantyhose an average of eight times.

Although you may spend a little more on the initial purchase for *graduated* support hose, with proper care they should have a longer life while still being cosmetically appealing.

If you are currently in treatment for vein disease, your health care provider may carry this type of stocking. The ones listed in the appendix do not require a prescription. Most of the listed manufacturers also make higher compression stockings, along with an array of other compression products, including a line for men. You can call the manufacturer for a local distributor. Note: Not all distributors will carry every product the manufacturer makes so you may have to ask what products are available. The distributor will probably have brochures and fabric swatches so you can choose products you want to order.

There are a few things you should note before comparing the various products:

- Lyrcra spandex (or spandex, a generic term) is usually found in more expensive hose. It is very stretchy, adding to comfort and fit, and helps prevent bagging (not a problem in any of the hose tested, even when going up a size to compensate for stockings that ran a little small).
- Nylon contributes to sheerness of the hose.
- Compression listing are for the amount of compression at the ankle. Ankle, calf, and thigh measurements will provide a better fit than height and weight measurements.
- With the exception of one manufacturer (Kelhart, Inc.), all prices listed are approximate because distributors set their own prices.
- When comparing comfort and fit, bear in mind that higher compression stockings may be more difficult to apply but provide better support.

Manufacturer	CAMP
Product Name	Airos
Fabric	85% nylon, 15% spandex
Available Colors	Nude, taupe, white, black, ivory, navy
Compression at ankle (in mmHg)	6-12
Maternity Sizes Available?	Yes*
Measurements needed	Height & weight
Number of sizes available	5
Sell direct to consumer?	No
How to order	Call 1-800-492-1088 for local distributor
Price range: Pantyhose/maternity	$21/$26
COMMENTS	*Maternity sizes available only in nude, taupe, white & black

Manufacturer	KELHART SYSTEMS, INC.
Product Name	Sheer Support
Fabric	Not available
Available Colors	Black, beige, white
Compression at ankle (in mmHg)	15
Maternity Sizes Available?	Yes
Measurements needed	Height & weight
Number of sizes available	5
Sell direct to consumer?	Yes
How to order	Call 1-517-487-0099 or fax 1-517-371-5564
Price range: Pantyhose/maternity	$13+ shipping
COMMENTS	VISA & MC orders accepted. Shipping discount given on order of multiple stockings

Manufacturer	BICOMPRESSION SYSTEMS, INC
Product Name	Venosan Legline 15
Fabric	75% nylon, 25% spandex
Available Colors	White, black, beige
Compression at ankle (in mmHg)	15
Maternity Sizes Available?	No
Measurements needed	Height & weight
Number of sizes available	5
Sell direct to consumer?	No
How to order	Call 1-800-888-0908 for local distributor
Price range: Pantyhose/maternity	$19/$43

COMMENTS

Manufacturer	JUZO
Product Name	LiteLine
Fabric	Spandex & nylon (% not available)
Available Colors	Champagne, hazel, slate & barely black
Compression at ankle (in mmHg)	15
Maternity Sizes Available?	Yes*
Measurements needed	Height & weight
Number of sizes available	6
Sell direct to consumer?	No
How to order	Call 1-800-222-4999 for local distributor
Price range: Pantyhose/maternity	Not available
COMMENTS	*Maternity sizes available only in champagne & barely black

Manufacturer	MEDI, U.S.A.
Product Name	OTC
Fabric	76% nylon, 24% spandex
Available Colors	Black, beige
Compression at ankle (in mmHg)	18
Maternity Sizes Available?	Yes
Measurements needed	Ankle, calf, thigh
Number of sizes available	4
Sell direct to consumer?	No
How to order	Call 1-800-633-6334 for local distributor
Price range: Pantyhose/maternity	$45-$50/$56-$60

COMMENTS

Manufacturer	BICOMPRESSION SYSTEMS, INC
Product Name	Venosan Legline 20
Fabric	75% nylon, 25% spandex
Available Colors	Black, grey, ivory, sahara
Compression at ankle (in mmHg)	20
Maternity Sizes Available?	Yes
Measurements needed	Height & weight
Number of sizes available	5
Sell direct to consumer?	No
How to order	Call 1-800-888-0908 for local distributor
Price range: Pantyhose/maternity	$36/$43

COMMENTS

Manufacturer	FREEMAN MFG. CO.
Product Name	Vena Flo Fashion 20
Fabric	65% nylon, 35% spandex
Available Colors	Black, beige, white
Compression at ankle (in mmHg)	20
Maternity Sizes Available?	Yes*
Measurements needed	Height & weight
Number of sizes available	5
Sell direct to consumer?	No
How to order	Call 1-800-253-2091 for local distributor
Price range: Pantyhose/maternity	$35-$55/$40-$65
COMMENTS	*Maternity available only in black & beige

Manufacturer	SIGVARIS
Product Name	Delilah
Fabric	80% nylon, 20% lycra
Available Colors	White, pearl, navy, taupe, beige, black,
Compression at ankle (in mmHg)	24
Maternity Sizes Available?	Yes
Measurements needed	Height & weight*
Number of sizes available	6
Sell direct to consumer?	No
How to order	Call 1-800-322-7744 for local distributor
Price range: Pantyhose/maternity	$20/$22
COMMENTS	*According to the mfr. this will be available with ankle, calf & thigh measurements (probable increase in price)

PHYSICIAN'S GUIDE TO ORDERING COMPRESSION

20-30 mm Hg: *For heaviness and fatigue in the legs... Mild varicosities without significant disposition for edema...Post sclerotherapy...Initial varices during pregnancy...Small varicose dialations of cutaneous veins...*

30-40 mm Hg: *Relief of aching heaviness and fatigue caused by varices...Post sclerotherapy...Post surgical stripping...Prophylaxis of Thrombosis...Prophylaxis and treatment of complications of varicose veins and post phlebitic syndrome with chronic venous insufficiency... Varices during pregnancy...Pregnant patients with previous phlebitis...Control of edema and effective scar formation after burns...Stasis dermatitis due to chronic venous insufficiency...*

40-50 mm Hg: *For severe degrees of above...Emphasized edema from above causes...Correctable lymphedema...Severe chronic venous insufficiency as with post phlebetic syndrome...Chronic venous problems after surgery...Venous ulcers...*
Contraindications: *High grade arterial insufficiency...Wet dermatoses...Cutaneous infections...Dermatitis in acute stage...*

✂Cut on dashed line

R℞ for Graduated Compression Support

Patient Name _____

Diagnosis _____

Physician's Signature _____

COMPRESSION	PANTY HOSE	MATERNITY	MEN'S LEOTARD
20-30 mm Hg			
30-40 mm Hg			
40-50 mm Hg			

FYI: Referral And Support Group Information

American College of Phlebology

for a referral to a physician in your area who specializes in venous disease write or call: 930 N. Meacham Rd., Schaumburg IL 60173 (847) 330-9830

web site: VeinsOnline.com

American Society of Phlebectomy

for a physician referral call 515-222-8346
web site: http://www.veindoctor.com

National Health Information Center

health information referral service 1-800-336-4797

Restless Leg Syndrome Foundation, Inc.

for information regarding their quarterly newsletter (*The Night Walker)* write to: RLSF, Inc., 304 Glenwood Ave., Raleigh NC 27603-1407

for local support group: write to: RLSF, Inc., Nat'l Support Group Co-ordinator, 10287 Silverado Circle, Bradenton FL 34202

web site: http://www.rls.org

Glossary

Artery: a blood vessel that conveys blood from the heart to any part of the body

Chronic venous insufficiency: a chronic condition of poor venous blood flow, swelling, and weakening of the skin tissue

Circulation: the continuous movement of blood through the heart and blood vessels, maintained chiefly by the action of the heart

Deep vein thrombosis (DVT): a condition in which a deep vein(s) is partially or totally blocked by a clot

Doppler ultrasound: a test used to diagnose blood clots or weak valves in the legs that uses ultrasound, sending high frequency sound waves which are reflected from moving red blood cells

Duplex imaging: a non-invasive procedure that analyzes blood flow and produces a visual image of the blood vessel

Invasive: requiring the entry of a needle, catheter, or other medical and especially surgical instrument into a part of the body for the purposes of diagnosing or treatment

Ligation: a surgical procedure during which the varicose vein(s) is tied off

Phlebitis: inflammation of a vein, often occurring in the legs and involving the formation of a thrombus, characterized by swelling, pain, and a change of skin color

Phlebology: the study of the anatomy, physiology and diseases of veins

Sclerotherapy: a treatment for varicose veins, hemorrhoids, and excessive bleeding in which blood flow is diverted and the veins collapsed by injection of a hardening solution

Stripping: a surgical procedure in which the varicose vein is removed

Superficial Vein: a vein close to the surface of the skin

Thrombus: a fibrinous clot that forms in and obstructs a blood vessel, or that forms in one of the chambers of the heart

Thrombophlebitis: the presence of a thrombus in a vein accompanied by inflammation of the vessel wall

Ulcer: a sore or break-down of the skin surface and/or deeper tissue

Ultrasound: sound waves which are transmitted over a blood vessel and reflect off of moving red blood cells

Valves: cup-like structures within the inner wall of a vein which prevent backward flow of blood

Varicose Veins: veins close to the surface of the leg which have become stretched and are bulging and uneven in appearance

Veins: blood vessels that carry the blood from the body back to the heart

Venous: relating to the vein or blood flow in the vein

Venous stasis ulcer: an open sore caused by severe or long term swelling of the leg, which weakens the skin tissue

Index

CPSIA information can be obtained at www.ICGtesting.com
Printed in the USA
LVOW07s0205210415

435339LV00002B/475/P